Fitness Professionals Guide to the NeuroRevolution

Dr. Eric Cobb

NOTICE OF COPYRIGHT & MEDICAL DISCLAIMER

1ST Edition January 2014
2nd Edition July 2014

DISCLAIMER

The information provided by Z-Health Performance Solutions, LLC ("Z-Health") is strictly intended for your general knowledge and for informational purposes only.

Z-Health shall not be responsible or liable for the content, use, information, or products and services of these resources. Additionally, Z-Health shall not be held responsible for the conduct of any company, website or individual mentioned in this product, associated websites, or any Z-Health Product.

You are encouraged to confirm any information obtained from or through this product or any Z-Health Product with other sources, and review all information regarding any medical condition or treatment with your physician. Should you have any healthcare-related questions, please call or see your physician or other healthcare provider immediately.

You should never disregard medical advice or delay in seeking it because of something you have read here or in any Z-Health Products. The opinions expressed in this publication represent the views of Z-Health Performance Solutions, LLC.

If you have questions, please contact: info@zhealth.net.

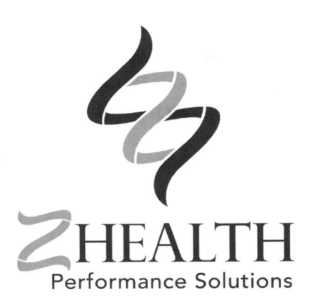

HEALTH

Performance Solutions

Table of Contents

Special Note

The following information I originally shared at NPE's Megatraining. After a number of Z-Health trainers found out about the presentation, they urged me to make the information more widely available and accessible to the personal trainers and other health and fitness professionals.

The best way to do that was to take the recording, have it transcribed and make it available for purchase. We've made every effort to edit the transcription and keep the message and context intact.

If you scroll to the end of the book, you will see a link to a private web page where you can access the original video and audio files at no additional cost. I'm making them available because I know that not everyone is a reader; some of you would rather enjoy watching a video or listening to just the audio. The private web page is there for you as a purchaser of this book. Enjoy!

Introduction

I will start by providing a little background on Z-Health Performance and myself. I talk in front of groups anywhere from 225 to 250 days a year. I teach multilevel certification programs all over the country.

I normally teach four- to six-day workshops. I do not ever use notes when teaching, so I tend to just start and go. My goal is to give you some takeaway tools and concepts to better point you in an effective direction from a marketing perspective.

Our company's marching orders, if you will, are based on the idea that we train the top one percent. If you want to be as good as you can be, you need systems to make that happen. That is why you are here (at NPE's Mega Training™). We cannot be good at everything, and so we need systems in place to help us to be good at the things that we are not so good at doing… or those things that are not our natural gift or unique ability.

What we are going to talk a lot about today is the brain. We are going to talk about neurology. Sean (with NPE) said something interesting on this subject. He said, "What they're doing is maybe 10 or 20 years ahead of what you're going to see currently in the business." I would say that is very accurate.

Filter Effect

How many of you have ever heard of the filter effect from research? Has anybody ever heard of the filter effect?

The filter effect says that what is happening in labs around the world right now is going to take approximately 15 years to filter down to the average field practitioner. This means that pain science as it currently stands is not being studied by your doctors.

Due to the filter effect, field practitioners do not know about recent developments in the field. Your physical therapists do not know about it. This filter effect also holds true when it comes to performance and changes in athletic performance, and to plyometrics. The research that is going right now that either proves or disproves what is currently popular will take 15 years to get down to the average practitioner.

From a business perspective, you should question why this is so. There are many ways you can use this idea to begin to differentiate yourself for the coming years in your profession. That is what I want to talk about today. I want to talk to you today about the field of Practical Neuroscience.

Practical Neuroscience is a weird field, but what is interesting is that if you look through academia right now, then you will see that neuroscience is a new, hot topic. Neuroscience actually is becoming sexy.

Your Brain Runs Your Body

The new technology of pain relief is relevant because your brain runs through your body. If you do not know how to manage the brain, then ultimately the body begins to create more and more issues for you. What we are looking for is a high-speed way to get stuff done.

I have a fairly strong academic background, but more importantly, I have an athletic background. Moreover, probably more important than all of that is the fact that I come from a strange history.

Why Z-Health?

I was one of those sick kids. I was born with a bunch of odd birth defects, and I spent my first two or three years in the hospital. I figured that I was going to die, and then over time, I apparently did not, and now I have made it this far in life. I had this weird blend of genetics. I had musculoskeletal problems as well as GI stuff and problems with my lungs and heart.

I believe my psyche enabled me to survive because from the earliest memories that I have, I was only interested in two things. I was interested in fitness and I was interested in fighting; that was it. The only things that I was ever interested in.

I read my first exercise book at the age of 5 years old. And, believe it or not, I read Gray's anatomy at the age of 11. I grew up in a small farm town in Mississippi and yet I had an intense interest in health and performance. Like I said, I have this weird blend of genetics. I started playing tennis and I got involved in martial arts. My athletic background led me to many interesting places in life. I have been all over the world competing, training and teaching. I am going to talk a lot about scientific developments, but you should understand that I am an athlete at heart. That is what I care about. I care about making people move.

Entrepreneur's Struggle

If you are an entrepreneur, then you know that your time is precious. You only get a short amount of time, and what's more important are the times when you are working with clients, and you only have a short amount of time to impress them.

You need to impress them; you need to create changes quickly. Ultimately, it is that quick change that assures them that you have great competence in your field.

Does anybody know who Dan Sullivan is? He runs a company called The Strategic Coach. This is probably one of my favorite quotes in the entire world.

"All progress begins by telling the truth."

There is a lot of information out there, and having invested hundreds of thousands of dollars in education. What I can tell you is that what Z-Health shares in our education programs is not what you get in other places. This is not because what we teach is not right or because it is not known, but because it is very difficult for people to apply some things practically unless you play with it a lot. All progress begins by telling the truth.

3 C Continuum

I am going to give you a three C continuum; these are three words that begin with the letter C.

The first word is clarity.

The second word is competence.

The third word is confidence.

Clarity, competence, and confidence: that is a continuum.

Clarity → Competence → Confidence

Unfortunately, what you see in the world are many people that actually start on the wrong end of this continuum. They try to start on the confidence end.

How many of you know people like that? They are very confident that they can accomplish anything. However, they do not have any real competence. Does everyone understand that?

Clarity

One of the things that I talk quite a bit about is that you need clarity in your life. What does clarity mean? It means that I have a very distinct definition of what I am doing, and that I know what I am trying to accomplish.

Another one of my favorite quotes is from my combative mentor, who I also used to work with, Tony Blauer. He is probably one of the smartest people in the world when it comes to dealing with violence. One of our favorite definitions that we used in teaching courses was this:

"The clarity with which we define something determines its usefulness."

In other words, if you cannot define it very well, then it may not be of much use to you. To help define things we have old journalism, which lists who, what, when, where, why, and how. In order to be better in your profession, you need to start defining things by asking a series of relevant questions, including asking yourself who your clients are, why are your clients coming into your office, and what are the unique services that you offer to potential clients?

Suppose that we go into any gym in the United States, and we look at anybody in that gym who has been training for more than a year. If you were to pull one of these people aside, a lot of them would tell you that the primary reason that they are in that gym is to change the way that they look. Isn't this correct? This is what I call naked mirror syndrome.

What do you want? You want to look better naked in the mirror. I am not saying that is a bad goal. I think that is a good thing, but how many people after two years of hard work have actually reached the physique goals that they began with? What do you think is the number of people that have achieved their fitness goals, percentage wise? Do you think that it is one percent, two percent, or even three percent?

What would you do if you had a laptop that only worked one percent of the time? You would throw it out. You would think, "You know what? This is a useless piece of equipment. Why do clients keep coming back for one percent success? Why do they keep paying good money to not accomplish what they say that they want to accomplish?"

You need to really think about these questions because the answer is that what your client says is not what they mean. This is the whole clarity discussion. Why are they there? Whenever you deal with human beings, they are very complex. They are a strange breed.

How many of you have ever heard of a metabolic word study?

Here is an example of how a metabolic word study is typically done. You tell your client,, "Okay, here is what is going to happen.In your program for the next 4-6 weeks you are going to take this journal. You are going to write down everything that passes your lips; everything that you eat and everything that you drink. You're going to write it all down."

Then, they go out and they live their lives, as they would normally do. The only exception is that they write it all down; they put it in their journal. At the end of that period, you will take them into this locked environment called the metabolic word, and you do not let them out.

You feed them exactly what they wrote down, and you can guess what happens. They all lose weight. This is because everybody lies. That is the thing. They are not doing it on purpose. They are not doing it because they want to lie, but because we have so many things that happen in our lives, and we just do it unconsciously.

Helping people to really understand why they are seeing you is extremely important, and it is more important for you because you are the one that is providing the service. You need clarity. Most people when they walk in the door tell you one thing, and what they really mean is that they just want to be better.

It takes a big step. Think about the people that walk through your door 40 or 50 pounds overweight and who haven't exercised in 20 years. Every time that they get up in the morning, they look in the mirror and they say, "God, what is wrong with me? Why can't I turn down this food? Why do I look like this?" They are asking themselves these questions all the time.

What you are providing them at the most basic level is hope. You are providing them hope that they can be different, and that they can change. Our job as high-level coaches is to not only provide them hope through being confident and encouraging, but to also help them to create change as fast as humanly possible. Does everyone understand that?

Ultimately, if you can do that, then you can differentiate your business from everyone else.

How many of you have clients that are in pain currently? Look around the room, everybody keep your hand up. That is a 100% hands up rate.

Pain, generally speaking, has been considered the realm of the doctor and the physical therapist for years. Guess what? Pain is the realm of the person that is experiencing it. That is what pain neuroscience now tells us. Pain is your responsibility. If you have it, then it is your responsibility. It is not anyone else's responsibility to get rid of it. All that they can do is to give you the path.

The hard part is that you have all of these people that want to be different. They want to move better, and they want to look better. How many athletes do we have in here? That is a trick question. Everybody should raise your hands. You all work out. You make your living with your body. Isn't that correct? By definition, you are all considered professional athletes.

How many of you have ever attempted to compete maybe in football, tennis, track, wrestling, or whatever? How many of you have ever tried to compete despite a physical injury? How did that work out for you? Although we like to say, "Oh yeah, I'm that guy. I will just push through. I'll just get through it, I'll be okay," we should realize that this is not true because you will not be able to do this: At least not for very long.

Hurt athletes typically sit on the bench. They quit playing. Eventually, they quit moving. If you look at the American College of Sports Medicine, you will learn that 85% of people in the United States that began an exercise program quit that exercise program within 6 weeks due to an injury, 85%.

Hopefully, we are not routinely seeing that, but a lot of those people are out there trying to train on their own. This means that you have a tremendous market of people who actually want to change, but they do not know how. 85% of the population to be exact. I like statistics.

When you look at the United States, does anyone have an idea of how many chronic exercisers there are? Chronic exercisers, by definition, are people that have exercised for one year or more regularly. What percentage of the United States population fits that definition? Does anybody know? 7% of the United States population is considered to fall into the chronic exerciser category, which is an unbelievably low number.

What does that tell you again about your business? It should tell you that there is plenty of money to be made, but once again, we have to show them that there is a path that clients can follow to achieve their goals. If I come back to my 3C continuum, this is the clarity part, and I could go on for days and days about the need for clarity in our professions.

Competence

How is competence relevant? You are here with a marketing course. You are looking at how to sell things better. You are asking yourself, "How do I market better?"

On this subject, ultimately all the speakers yesterday said the same thing, to some degree. You had better be your own billboard. You had better look the part, but more importantly, you need to have the integrity to act the part. However, you can fake it, kind of.

One of my favorite sayings with fighters, because I work a lot with professional fighters, is that you cannot fake endurance in the ring. Well, you really cannot fake competence for very long either. You can act as if you have it all together, but there is nothing that builds unshakeable confidence in your capacity to help people like having great, relevant skill sets.

Confidence

During Sean's talk yesterday, he said that the number one place to invest your money is in yourself. What was he talking about there? He was telling us to build competence because the more time that you spend building competence, the greater your confidence. It is a simple, easy to remember continuum.

You need to know who you are. You need to know who they are. You need to have the skill sets to help them no matter what is going on in your business. And, from all of that you can now speak with tremendous confidence because you can provide them with exactly what they need. This makes the sales process much, much easier.

Differentiation is the next thing that I am going to talk about, and then I will actually talk about some hopefully cool science related stuff. I put a brain up here because one of the things that you want to start thinking about is the person that you are today as well as the person that you are going to be in the next 5 years.

This may sound like silly, cliché, self-help stuff. Who are you today? Who are you going to be in the next 5 years? It really is not. This is probably the most critical question that you can ask yourself. Here is what we know about neurology at this point. The human brain is a target-seeking system. It is a target-seeking system and the way that it seeks out its target is very interesting.

For instance, if I take this pen and throw it down on the floor, there are innumerable paths that I can take to actually pick up the pen. I could walk around this way. I could dive over, do a flip, then pick it up. I could even get down there to pick it up with my teeth. What is interesting is that your brain, whenever you give it a target, goes through this computational sequence. There is a whole science in mathematics called Bayesian mathematics or Bayesian theory. What has been happening over the last 15 years is that people have been trying to build robots and neural networks that function like the human brain.

Secret to Getting Good

If you want to get good at something, then you should look at people outside your own industry. This is one of the things that we do all the time within Z-Health. We are continually asking the question , "What are people outside the health care industry doing that can help elucidate who we are as well as what we are supposed to be doing a little bit better?"

For the last 10 years or so, I have been doing a lot of study in the whole development of neural networks and robotics because what they are trying to do is they are trying to build these machines that act like us. This means that there is a very intense programming process that they have to go through. In order to do that, they have to understand more about how we actually work. One of the mathematicians currently working in this field is Emmanuel Todorov; he is from the University of California Santa Barbara, and he is currently working at the University of Washington.

The Brain Equation

These mathematicians, including Emmanuel Todorov, are trying to come up with something comparable to the $E=MC^2$ equation for the human brain. They are trying to determine how the human brain actually works as well as discover the one equation that will explain how the human brain functions. What they did is they built this test and these models; they kept trying to run simulations against what we know about how the human mind seems to function. Ultimately, in that long process, they incorporated this mathematical theory called Bayesian theory into their study. Bayesian theory is actually from the field of economics.

Years ago, Bayesian theory was applied to look at the economies of nations. The whole idea was to determine if we could use a mathematical equation to figure out certain probabilities, such as what is going to happen with the economy on the national level. You have to think about this carefully. Researchers started doing these studies and they went, "Look, this is weird. The human brain appears to function according to the law of probabilities."

In other words, whenever I throw that pen down to the floor, my brain has innumerable options that it can choose from to retrieve it. Basically, what it does is that it looks forward, and it determines the probabilities; it then tries to choose what, hopefully, is the most efficient and best option in order to help me to accomplish the task.

Without a Target, It's Hard to Aim

Who you are today and who you are 5 years from now is not an idle question because if you do not give your brain a target, then it is hard to aim and achieve a desirable outcome. That is how your brain functions. If you do not have a target, then it is hard to aim. There is no way to come up with probabilities. I can take a dart and admit that I have no idea where the target is, so I will just toss it out there and hope for the best. However, it is not desirable to live your day-to-day life in this manner.

For example, your business right now is what it is. 5 years from now, it will be what it will be based off of how well you differentiate yourself from everyone else. I think that is an easy concept to understand.

In marketing terms, we call the process of differentiation branding or brand awareness. At the end of the day, how you differentiate yourself will make all the difference. I think that everybody who is in the fitness industry as well as everybody who is in the health care industry who is really in this entrepreneurial mindset is headed in the direction of the brain and the nervous system. I will give you a little bit more shape to this in just a second. Let's move on a little.

Introduction to Neuroplasticity

Have you ever heard the term neuroplasticity? If you have, then that is good. If you are thinking about reading any book this year to advance your career, then you need to read "The Brain that Changes Itself." Some of you may disagree with me because there are other great marketing books, but ultimately when you read this you are going to look at yourself differently in the mirror. Do you remember Sean's number one rule, which is the core value of NPE? He states that the number 1 core value is personal responsibility. If you read this book, "The Brain that Changes Itself," then all of the sudden you are going to go, "Holy cow, he's right. I am responsible for becoming who I am."

Dr. Norman Doidge wrote the book "The Brain that Changes Itself." Dr. Doidge writes a lot about neuroplasticity. Let me just give you a broad definition of what neuroplasticity is. Since 1995, the whole science of understanding the brain has changed. In fact, many neuroscientists now will tell you that 80% of what we thought that we knew in 1995 about how the human brain functions is wrong. Our understanding of who you are as people as well as how you function has changed unbelievably because we have obtained new technologies. Probably the most important one is called a functional MRI.

A functional MRI along with Transcranial Magnetic Simulation (TMS) allows us to look at your brain while you are doing things to see how it works. Ultimately, what we are discovering is that we can map the brain. Therefore, when a subject is experiencing an emotion, we can take a picture of the brain, including the parts of the brain that are functioning to determine the subject's emotions, such as if they are happy, if they are sad, et cetera.

Dr. Bach-y-Rita was an early pioneer in neuroplasticity. Dr. Bach-y-Rita was a medical maverick. He had been through multiple residencies. He never did things in a normal way. One day, his father had a massive stroke. In other words, he was almost vegetative. He lost all motor function, and he lost the ability to speak. His dad was a teacher at, I believe, City University of New York.

In the book, "The Brain that Changes Itself," the neurologist says to Dr. Bach-y-Rita, "Listen, he is what he is. There is no improvement from here." Despite receiving this discouraging news from the attending neurologist, Dr. Bach-y-Rita took his dad back to Mexico because he has the personality that says, "Well, that may be true and it may not be true. However, we should still be able to do something for him."

By taking his dad back to Mexico, Dr. Bach-y-Rita started this very early version of what has now become known as neuro-developmental therapy. He realized that it was alright at that point if his dad was like a baby who really had no body control. This just made him interested in learning how to determine how a baby begins to learn to move. First, Dr. Bach-y-Rita started trying to make his dad grasp stuff as well as to make him move his mouth and move his tongue. He was teaching him how to do all of these somewhat basic things.

Over the course of 2 years, his dad regained almost full function. His dad went back to teaching and living on his own. It was a miraculous recovery. A number of years later, his dad passed away. At this point you must realize that Dr. Bach-y-Rita was a real scientist because they did an autopsy on his dad, and when he looked at his dad's brain with the pathologist they saw that was the stroke that his dad had experienced was huge. It was enormous.

We have a motor cortex that gives commands from the brain down into the body. Dr. Bach-y-Rita father's stroke had actually destroyed all of the motor cortex except for 3% of all the descending motor control systems. There was no way according to standard medical science that he could have recovered even the tiniest particle of all the movement that he recovered under Dr. Bach-y-Rita's highly individualized care. Dr. Bach-y-Rita, after this experience with his Dad, said, "You know what, I think the brain can change."

The Brain Can Change

How many of you believe that the brain can change? This belief puts you in a small minority because up until about 10 years ago, it was believed, particularly in the medical profession, that the brain was fixed after the age of about 25 years old. It was commonly thought by medical professionals that the brain did not change after that arbitrary milestone. They believed that all of the tracks were built in, they were hard-wired, and you were who you were. However, nothing could be further from the truth.

Dr. Bach-y-Rita realized, "You know what, that's pretty interesting that Dad was able to recover all of this stuff, so the brain must be able to change. Therefore, if I can teach a man with no motor control to move again, then I bet that I could teach blind people to see. I bet that I could teach deaf people to hear." And, this is precisely what he accomplished in the field.

He started with blind people. He built a chair and on top of the chair, he put a camera. That camera digitized information and that information was sent into a strip of plastic imbedded with little electrodes that ran down the back of the chair.

If you have had a TENS unit on or something similar before, you have experienced a little bit of a shock. However, Dr. Bach-y-Rita said, "I bet we could transmit information into the skin of the back, and if the brain is capable of what we think it is capable of, then it will learn to adjust." Through his work, this is precisely what happened.

Over a period of training, the participants began to see using the skin of their back. Because what is interesting about the human brain is that when you tell it to do something repeatedly, it is wired to do just that. The human brain is trainable.

That is why so many of you have a much greater opportunity to be successful than your peers because you are here telling your brain to do things that your colleagues are not doing. You are investing the time and you are investing the energy in becoming better at your profession.

The device that Dr. Bach-y-Rita developed was called the brain port. He figured that people do not want to sit in the chair and just see. Instead, they want to move around so he started developing and miniaturizing the brain port.

Seeing with the Tongue

They changed the brain port a little bit because they realized that it was cumbersome to have these strips on the back. They decided that they were going to use a strip of plastic on the tongue. There are blind people out there right now that are walking around with a little camera on a strap and a belt unit like a microphone with a little plastic tube that runs up. They can slip that piece on their tongue, and they can see the world.

They have actually developed this technology to the point right now that they can recognize faces. That is how good this specialized device works with the tongue. That is the capability of your brain. You have to understand that this is the science right now.

Your brain is capable of amazing things. You are capable of amazing things. However, the challenge is to make sure that your brain is continuously focused on change. You have to begin to focus on the change that you want. As I said without a target, it is tough to aim and achieve desirable results.

You need to read this book, "The Brain that Changes Itself." As I said, it will change your perspective of yourself, and more importantly, of what it is possible to achieve in your daily lives. Again, we will go back to our clarity, competence, and confidence discussion.

Every Problem is a Brain Problem

Every time that you start to get frustrated with a client who is not making a change, you should remember this and you will go, yeah, we're not rewiring your brain quite right. Everything that happens in the body is about rewiring the brain, and making it run more efficiently.

How many of you have clients that struggle with their dietary plan? I am certain that no one in here has ever struggled with his or her own dietary plan. That is a brain problem. It is not a self-discipline problem. It is not a willpower problem, but it is a brain problem. Everything is a brain problem.

There is a lot of material that you need to understand about how the brain functions. Everyone is an athlete; it is important to me that you start to recognize that as well as the fact that everything is a skill. Because whenever you watch the Z-Health training session, you are going to see many people doing things, which will make you think, "That's weird. Why do you have that old lady doing vision stuff? Why is that older lady doing something like playing catch? Why is she warming up?" We treat everybody the same way; we assume that you are an athlete. You are a human being; therefore, you should be an athlete.

Many people get into the fitness industry or become fitness athletes because they cannot do anything else. Does everyone hear that? Many of your clients would rather be playing volleyball. They would rather play basketball, but maybe they cannot because they cannot see, or maybe because they have a balance problem. There are easy ways to assess these potential issues and fix them.

It is important to me that you start to understand these points: Everyone is an athlete, and the second thing, everything is a skill. I hope that you understand that second concept right now. You can all understand that marketing is a skill, and that closing is a skill. Is closing the same thing as writing a marketing piece? No, they are different.

Everything is a skill. When you look at moving and becoming stronger, more flexible, and having better range of motion, all of those are actually independent skills. Therefore, as a coach, you have to have great clarity about what your clients need the most. I am going to move on a little bit because this will help you to understand the brain a little bit more. We will now address a very simple question. Is the body more oriented towards survival or performance?

The Brain is Hard-Wired

How do you think that you are wired? You are wired for survival; you are not wired for high performance. How do we know that? Because if you throw something at me, I will flinch. If I touch a hot stove, then I will jerk my hand back. However, there is no such thing as a dunk reflex. I wish that there were, but there is not. There is no going fast reflex. Instead you get back, move away, and flinch. This is called a flexor withdrawal reflex. Whenever something really scares you, what do you do? You get small, you get tight, and you assume the fetal position so that none of the important parts located on the midline are eaten.

We are wired for survival more than for anything else. And, what is interesting is that if you understand that, then all of the sudden the problems that your clients have become much more accessible to you. I have this great picture to demonstrate this, hopefully you can see that. What we have there is synchronized flinching. It is a new Olympic sport.

A baseball bat is flying into the crowd at a baseball game is a perfect example of neurologic hard wiring. All the "victims" in this photo are doing the same thing. Even the arm angles and the facial expressions are all the same.

This is what you look like when a cat scares you when you are taking the trash out at night and you are thinking "Whoa," and then you try to look cool like it did not happen. That is who you are at the most basic level. You are a survival-based organism, so your brain is constantly going through probabilities, and it is constantly trying to decide if something is scary or not.

Your behavioral imperative is that you stay alive and not understanding this is a huge disconnect. I am going to talk a little bit about pain here in just a second. However, the thing that you need to realize is that all pain, all performance at the physical level, is governed by this. Your client's body is constantly deciding whether the activity that it is undergoing is dangerous or not.

That is what the body does. It is trying to determine if this proposed activity is scary or not. If it is too scary for the nervous system, then guess what it is going to do? It is going to try to make you **stop that activity.** It is a really simple idea. However, how it begins to manifest itself is pretty strange.

I had to put that picture up because that is a perfect example of the behavioral imperative. This is from one of our training courses. You can see that the guy is flinching. As danger increases, our instinctive responses go up.

How many of your clients have problems with their nutritional issues? One factor that is most strongly related to a behavioral imperative is the command to not starve oneself. The human nervous system tends to consider hunger as dangerous.

Many times, in the deep dark recesses of our mind, when our clients are following their diet plan we are thinking, "You lazy son of a gun." when we should say , "Oh, so you are just scared of starving." That is a productive attitude to have, and it begins to help you to frame things differently as well as to speak to people differently on this issue.

I am trying to give you relevant knowledge about how to differentiate your business. Ultimately, differentiating your business is based off competence and understanding things, which other people do not understand right now.

I am going to give you a physical example here in just a second because I am a movement guy, so I like for people to actually experience stuff rather than just hear about it. Right now, what you are seeing is what we understand about the danger assessment response in the field of neurology. .The human brain responds two ways to perceived threats.

The Natural Response Filter

The human brain's two response methods are called the low road and the high road. What I love about this is that it tells me that people are more alike than they think. We tend to believe that we are very rational people and make decisions based on this premise. However, we do not realize that we are wired to choose the low-road response.

Whenever you look at the human brain, there is this whole, strange wiring system. Nevertheless, what you need to understand is this. Everything that happens in your life, every single experience that you have in your life, passes through a filter.

That filter works down at the center of your brain in a part of the brain called the amygdala. Does anyone know the term binary? Binary is a system of computer codes comprised of zeroes and ones. The amygdala operates on a binary system. It takes in every bit of information from your environment including every thought that you have, every interaction with your client, everything that you experience physically; and it determines whether something is dangerous or not. That is its only job in the beginning, and that is defined as the low-road response.

The low-road response is three to four times faster than your conscious thinking. This means that you are going to respond reflexively before you respond logically at the most basic level.

This has huge implications in decision-making, as well as in sports. It has huge implications in the study of pain management as well as how we train people. Therefore, the ramifications are huge. Remember that you can have a low-road response and you can have a high-road response. The low road response is much faster, and it is much more direct. It tries to make you change your behavior.

This is a really old drawing. This dude is naked by the fire and I do not know why. I have tried multiple times to figure it out but I cannot and I do not recommend this behavior. If you can see the picture, then what you see is not only is he naked but he stuck his foot in the fire for some unknown reason.

There is a line that is leaving his foot; it is going up the leg, and up the back. Can you see up in the head? There is actually a little labeled dot. Can you see that? I will put the arrow up here. That is the label dot, the F.

This drawing was done in 1667, and it illustrates the Descartes reflex. What is interesting is that most of your therapists, doctors, and your clients all believe that this is how pain works. Everybody tends to believe that the brain is isolated. We have all heard about the right brain, left brain theory, which states that the right brain is for creativity, and that the left brain is for logic. You have the language center, you have the auditory center, and you have the visual center. However, all of that is wrong. The brain is much more fluid. It is much more complex.

Unfortunately, what happens is that people look at this simplistic idea of pain and they think that if they can just figure out the one solution, then their shoulder pain will go away. By knowing the underlying reason, knee pain will go away. They will get stronger or they will get faster because there is one answer for everything. There is not one answer for everything.

There are multiple answers, and if you understand this fact better, then it makes more sense. You must understand that pain does not work this way. There is no one, pain center in the brain. Unfortunately this 400-year-old pain theory is what most of your professionals are still operating with; that is a little longer than the 15-year filter effect. That is the 400-year filter effect.

With this in mind, we are going to go a little bit deeper because I need you to understand pain. Pain is a metaphor for a lot of stuff that you are talking about here for your business and everything else.

What has occurred over the last 15 years is that a brand new understanding has developed. Looking again at these pictures, that foot in the far corner of the picture has a tack underneath the toe. In other words, someone is stepping on something sharp. Then you see a routing through this nerve, which is traveling exactly like the Descartes reflex. The biggest difference occurs when you get up to the brain. What do you see there? You see multiple arrows.

The Threat NeuroMatrix

Here is what we now understand about what is happening. When someone is experiencing pain, if we take a picture of their brain at that moment, you do not see one area of the brain light up, but rather you see seven areas of the brain light up. What is really fascinating is that when you look at these different areas of the brain that light up and what they are generally associated with, they are not what you would expect. The areas of the brain that light up have more to do with things like the future and the past. They include thoughts like, "Have I hurt that knee before? Oh, yeah god, that feels the same. Oh geez, man, I blew my ACL 20 years ago."

Very little of the pain experience has to do with the actual physical injury. Instead, it questions what is this injury going to do to my work, my job and to my family? Your brain will also note how scary the experience is. You will note all of these different things.

What is cool about understanding this is that all of a sudden you begin to realize that you have greater control over all the stuff for yourself and your clients than you ever imagined, but it all comes down to whether you can understand it. We call this the Threat Neuromatrix in Z-Health.

There is a very simple reason for that. Let me ask you a simple question. How many of you have a chronic "thing?" It can be a shoulder, a hip, a knee, a headache, or whatever. If you are honest, then you should raise your hand at some point because you are an athlete.

Athletes in general have something, "Oh, yeah it's my trick knee." Really?, What kind of trick does it do? Rolls over, bark sometimes? I do not know. "It's my bad shoulder." What did it do that made it so bad? Ultimately, what happens is that you get better at what you practice.

Let's say that you are 20 years old and you go out and play in a soccer game. While playing, you roll your ankle, and then you spend 6 weeks hobbling around on a sore ankle. You have now built a nice pain pattern, so that whenever there is a threat, and you should remember that we are governed by threat, your body will very often go...I want you to quit this relationship that you are in, but it cannot really get your attention that way. Therefore, what does it try to do?

It tries to get your attention any way that it can. Very often, it will get your attention by making what used to hurt, hurt again because it is easy for the mind to just succumb to pain. Does everyone understand that? Let me give you a better example, maybe a different example. In 1993, they did this huge study at Boeing. The Boeing study took 3,000 people, and the researchers studied the participants for about 18 months. The whole idea was to figure out who was going to develop lower back pain.

Who Is Going To Develop Back Pain?

They did all of these biometrics in order to determine the likelihood of developing lower back pain. They weighed them. They did strength testing on them. They did flexibility testing on them. They looked at their job requirements, and they asked them a series of questions, including whether they sit or stand for long periods, and whether they routinely moved stuff around in their day-to-day lives. They were trying to determine what exactly the participants did on a daily basis.

They got the data together over a period of 18 months. They collated it, and they put it together in order to draw conclusions. There was one factor but only one factor that they came up with that was a good indicator of who was going to experience lower back pain.

Remember, lower back pain is the classic human experience. Has anybody here ever had it? Statistically, 80% to 90% of the US population is going to have a bad episode at some point. One factor is a determinant of lower back pain… do you want to venture a guess as to what it was?

The actual answer that they came up with was job dissatisfaction. How much do you hate your job?

If you hate your job, then you can get lower back pain.

If you hate your life, then you can get shoulder pain, or whatever other ailments.

One hundred percent of you raised your hands when I asked the question "how many of you have clients with pain". When you begin to understand this stuff, then what happens is that you go all the way back to the clarity concept. What do they want? They want to be better. They want a different life. Therefore, a lot of the pain that they experience is something that you are going to take care of just by giving them hope, just by giving them direction, and just by giving them a plan.

There are many ways to take care of a client and their issues quickly. Whenever we start talking about the threat neuromatrix, we try to boil things down to a more physical level because we are not counselors, and we are not psychologists. At the end of the day, I always tell people that I am a fighter and that I am a practical guy.

How many of you grew up in the Bruce Lee era? Bruce Lee was one of my boyhood heroes. One of my favorite sayings ever was when someone asked him to define a true martial art. He smiled and responded, "When fist meets flesh."

I do not care how things get done, but that is the whole idea. We are very practical. I am giving you all this theoretical stuff. Let me give you some very practical stuff now to start thinking about. I am going to talk about what has been called the threat hierarchy.

The Performance and Threat Hierarchy

Your entire life is an environmental interaction. You are either interacting with your internal environment or your external environment? Do you understand that?

Let's say that I am out for a run. I am out on the pavement jogging along when I look up and there is my neighbor with his Rottweiler. I hate that dog, and I am running. Then I look up and the dog is going nuts for whatever reason. It sees me and maybe we feel the same way about one another. He is digging around and my brain is doing what? It is assessing probabilities for the given situation. Does my neighbor look capable of holding on to this animal, or should I turn around and go the other way. All of that information is being run through three primary filters: my visual system, my vestibular system, which is also known as my balance system that determines how I interact with gravity, and then my somatosensory or my proprioceptive system, which is my movement system. Does everyone understand that? You have three important systems in the body, which are defined as the visual, the vestibular, and the proprioceptive.

What happens if you somehow come to develop a deficit in any one of these systems? What do you think that will do to your performance? Is it going to hurt it, or is it going to improve it? What is very fascinating about this process is that it is actually hierarchical.

If I am trying to survive this encounter with the dog, then is it better that I see it early or is it better if I experience it physically? I would like to know what is coming in advance. That is your visual system. The visual system is your primary system. It is actually easy to assess, and it is very easy to train.

The Visual System

Do you understand that vision is a skill; that it is a learned skill? Most people say, "Oh, vision, yeah, yeah I got great eyes, 20/20," It is important to realize that the assertion that you have 20/20 vision has almost nothing to do with anything.

In sports you may have a great basketball player or a great tennis player. And, what do they say? Well, that athlete will say that he has great eyes, and that he has great vision. What does that mean?

There are nine different vision skills that you can test and that you can train. If you are not doing that, then you are not dealing with the number one threat to your clients. What will blow your mind is that you will start to discover that people have shoulder pain a lot of times not because their shoulder is screwed up, but because their vision is screwed up.

What would you do with your head and neck if you could not see? If I found myself in this situation, then I would try to get closer and try to adjust my head and neck position. My corrected posture would take care of my eyes. What are you going to do to the nerve that is going into your shoulders? Potentially, this is going to create a problem, but ultimately that is giving you a biomechanical answer to a neurologic problem because just having a visual problem is enough to make the world scarier. Does everyone understand that? The term that I gave you was a threat neuromatrix where everything comes down to threat perception. If my body wants me to survive, then it is more important for me to sit on my butt than it is for me to get up and move.

This is true for a lot of your clients. You ask them when you take initial history, "hey do you like sports?" And, your client replies, "I hate sports. I never was picked when I was a kid. The first time that I went out to play softball, I was hit on the face. I have hated sports ever since then. I'm just not athletic."

The truth is probably not that you are not athletic, you probably just cannot see. Wouldn't parents rather take their kids to the doctor than have them sit at home? No, they would not. In 2004, the US Olympic team did a survey to determine how many of its athletes had ever had an eye exam. The answer was that only 50% of the US Olympic team had had an eye exam at some point in their lives. That is our Olympic team. There is so much going on just for the visual system.

If you want something to differentiate your business, then you should realize that there are probably not many people that are making advances in this field. Not many people have heard about sports vision therapy. Nike was an exception to this. Sports vision is not just for athletes who are out there running around the track and playing football. It is for everybody that is in pain because vision always makes a difference.

The Vestibular System

Next you have the vestibular system. The vestibular system is your onboard balance system. It is what keeps you oriented within the environment. It is important to remember that the visual system and the vestibular system work together. You can test and train the vestibular system too.

Right now, we have many people out there who are doing what they think is balance training and vestibular work. They are BOSUing and wobble boarding, but what is interesting is that the vestibular system does not really respond very well to those types of activities.

I go into gyms all the time, and I often think, "is it a gym, or is it a circus event? " I am not sure that standing on a BOSU, juggling medicine balls, or whatever else that they are doing is really practical for most people. It is fun, and I am not saying not to do it if you enjoy it, but I am saying that if you are doing it for the wrong reason, then it is bad science number one, and it is not creating the results that you want. number two. You should look at all the research and you should determine if it really makes your balance better. When you stand on something that wobbles, then you only become good at standing on something that wobbles; that is it. Instead, you should focus on what makes you better standing on your feet.

What is interesting is that the vestibular system is designed to respond to head movement. What do people do as soon as they stand on something that wobbles? They keep their heads still. They are not really training to do what they think that they are training to do.

This is one of my favorite sayings ever,

"A bad idea embraced by millions upon millions of people is still a bad idea."

That entire training paradigm was created for one thing and one thing only and it has been completely warped. You do not need it. There are many things that you can do, and as I said if you enjoy it, then cool, you should keep it as the dessert of the program. However, you should realize that it is not the main course of the program. We want to be people who are working on what people need in their daily lives.

The Proprioceptive System

Finally there is the proprioceptive system, which is part of the movement system. This is what we are known for at Z-Health.

Let me ask you a simple question. Let's do a test. Everybody sit nice and tall. You do not have to stand up; you can just sit. We all have a neck. Some of you have worked out more than I have, so you have less of one, and I probably hate you for it at some level. I do not have traps, but here we go.

We are going to do a quick test. The human neck can move in a bunch of different directions, so let's do a test rotation first. Everyone just rotate … fantastic you all passed. Now, go back to the middle position. Now tilt … well done. Everybody act like a chicken … now forward and back, cool. You are doing pretty well so far. How about trying this one now? Alright and that is about a 3% pass rate on that one.

Then, can we start to combine them? Can you tilt, glide, and do all these different movements? Can you do that with every body part?

Can you move your neck?

Can you move your shoulder?

Can you move your wrist?

Can you move your hand, fingers, and spine? Can you do it?

Because if you cannot do these basic movements, then guess what? Your movements are not as good as they could be. What I tell people over and over again is to listen. Has anybody here ever traveled overseas? A few of you have. When I sold my practice years ago, I moved to Italy because I always wanted to live in Italy.

I moved to Florence where I went into practice with a friend just two days a week. He was working with the Italian Olympic team. We had the volleyball team; we had a cyclist and a couple of other groups. Within three days of moving to Italy, I was working with these athletes. I spoke no Italian. However, I had done the little Berlitz like book on the plane over to Italy; I actually had to learn Italian on the fly. Fortunately I am pretty good with languages and I pick them up fairly quickly.

Three months later, you could not tell that I did not speak good Italian in the clinic because I could talk about the body, movement, and all of that stuff. I was even told I had a nice Florentine accent. Then, I had to move, and I am on the phone with a real estate agent saying, "What is the word for kitchen?" I grabbed my dictionary, realizing that I had a really specific vocabulary.

Movement Fluency

I had a survival vocabulary for my environment. Guess what people have in terms of movement? They have a survival vocabulary of movement and nothing else. As a result, every time that they are confronted with a problem that they cannot solve, their natural threat response makes them stop. Does everyone understand? It is how we are wired.

At the most basic level, from this movement perspective, Z-Health begins our programs with the question … can you move every joint through every range of motion and can you control it? Once you have those skills, all of a sudden you see massive performance gains.

Generally, the people that start our program start hitting PRs in strength, speed, power after 4-6 weeks, and sometimes immediately. We have tons and tons of stories. We are very well known in the industry for immediate pain relief and immediate performance enhancements … where is Jason?

He came up to me yesterday. He walked up. He says, Doc, he starts moving the shoulder around. I saw him a few months ago in Chicago. He had 5 years of shoulder pain. However, within 3 minutes of drills, he tells me that his shoulder pain is gone.

I love the fact that we can help people quickly, but I am in for this for the long haul; the lifelong education process. What you are going to see is that you can build tremendous confidence in people by demonstrating competence, and nothing breeds confidence faster than helping people to get out of pain. Does everyone hear that?

Do you want a way to differentiate your business? I am not telling you to be a doctor; I am not telling you to be a therapist. However, I am telling you that if you do the basics and understand it, then all of a sudden, you will be able to do things that no one else can do and do them in a safe way.

There are many other directions that we can go with all of this stuff, but what I want you to think about right now is the importance of the visual system. Is it trainable, yes or no? That all sounds great in theory, but you have to know how to do it.

The vestibular system is the same way. The proprioceptive system is the same way.

Let me go onto the next slide here. I am just going to give you a quick rundown of all this stuff. As I said, vision is much more than 20/20. You have nine different elements that apply in sports.

How many of you would like to be better at training or you would like your trainers to be better at training? What I am trying to tell you is that if you begin to understand all this stuff, then you will be in a position within your business that will definitively differentiate you.

The Future of the Fitness Industry

The next 10 to 15 years, we are going to see a title shift in the fitness industry. I do not know how many of you follow this stuff politically. Right now you work in the most unregulated industry in history. It is unbelievable. How many personal trainers are there in the United States? There are approximately 125,000 trainers, and most of them have a certain type of certification. We have a good friend that runs a certification program in California. Two years ago, he did a documentary, and what he did is he went to a graveyard, and he pulled names off tombstones. Then he got those people certified.

You are here at a high-level event (or you are reading this book) for entrepreneurs, so I know that you are not one of those people I know that you are investing in yourself, and that you are investing in your skills all the time. In the coming years, you absolutely have to become focused on the fact that just because the personal training industry seems easy, does not mean that it is easy - although you get to wear sweats to work. The amount that you are charging your clients makes this profession really attractive, especially when you can begin charging after a 3 day certification process.

Ensure Your Success

This industry is going to shift into a wellness model. The people that have the highest level of education with the highest skill sets, and the people with the best capacity to demonstrate immediate results are the ones who are going to make all the money in this new system. It is going to actually divide further than it ever has before, and it is all going to be based off of neurology because I guarantee that you cannot get into a field of medicine anymore where neurology is not the key component in the field. Physical therapy along with everything else is shifting in this direction. As I said, what you are trying to do in your business is put yourself in a position to do more, and to create better results.

Whether you attend Z-Health Certification courses or not, at some level, you need to start incorporating the visual system, the vestibular system, and the movement system into your practice because all of these fields of study are important. All of them can be trained. All of them can be changed. As you get deeper into this, you will realize that I am not just dealing with an athlete here. I am dealing with everybody in pain, everybody with performance issues and everybody who is looking for quick results.

Threat Neuromatrix Demonstration

Now, I am going to talk about proprioception. I need a volunteer from the audience. Come on over. What is your name? Alex, I want to thank you for volunteering to do this. Do you mind taking your shoes off? I do not think that he is going to need this … this one. Has anybody here done MAT or muscle activation technique? A few of you have. We are going to do a quick muscle test on him. I just want to see how strong he is. Did you work out this morning?

Alex: "No."

Eric: "Good, lay on your back for me."

You may want to stand up so that you can see. I want you to just go up here and put your head over that way. What we are going to do … are you comfortable?

We are going to test a couple of different muscles in his body because I want to give you some examples of what we are talking about. Stretch your legs out for me.

The first test that I am going to do is on a muscle called gluteus medius. It is the hip muscle; you should make sure that your pelvis stays stable when you walk. If you try to do any kind of overhead pressing, and can't because of shoulder pain, then a lot of times it is this muscle that is creating the problem.

You need to understand kinetic chain theory as well as how the legs work for the arms. We are going to see how his gluteus medius is working so the test looks like this.

Go ahead and push out toward them as hard as you can, push, push, push. That is actually really good. He is very, very strong.

Push out. Nice.

What is interesting is that when you understand neurology, you start to understand the importance of the movement. I already showed you this.

Can you do all of the different neck movements? But, can you do that with your feet, your hands, and your back, et cetera? I am asking you to do this because sometimes there is a problem, somewhere, and right now, I am just going to his foot, and I am going to create a problem in order to demonstrate this. Is everyone okay with that?

What I am going to do is I am going to take one of the joints in his foot, and I am going to jam it. In other words, I am going to compress it just like that. That is all that there is to it. Did that hurt? No. I am going to retest him. Push out; push out. I wish that he would try harder, that would be good. This is a very different feeling.

Alex: "That's it man?"

Eric: "Nope, not without charging a great deal."

Alex: "That's a money maker."

Eric: "Actually, I'm going to fix this because I want to show you one other thing. "

What you are just seeing is that joint problems or joint immobility anywhere in the body can create muscular deficits. Does everyone understand that? Because the muscles respond neurologically to what the joints are telling them to do. If we open this joint back up, then he should be able to push out again ... that's actually really good. It surprised me because when you first test a lot of people, these muscles are very inhibited. His were not, which was good. Now, I am going to show you the really weird part as well as why whenever we deal with all this stuff that we deal with at Z-Health we are very comprehensive.

You can move your feet just like you move your neck because I can give you the same drills that we just did for the neck for your feet. There are similar versions for the feet because the feet have to be mobile. Nevertheless, every joint in the body has a potential to be negative. Let me show you this quickly.

This is his thumb. I am going to do the same thing to his thumb that I just did to his foot. I just took the thumb, and I jammed it together. He is going, "That was really weird." Go and push out again, again, hard, hard, hard.

What do you think happened? I am going to make it simple for you. You can stay there for just a sec, and we will fix you right up.

I said earlier that the brain is governed by threat. Does everyone remember that? When you have a lousy map of movement you just have your survival movement map, which makes it harder for your brain to predict outcomes for you.

It makes it harder for your brain to understand the directions that you are going to move, how you are going to create power, and how you are going to create strength. There is a lot of complicated stuff going on in that. Does that make sense to you, though?

If your joints are a problem, then your vision is a problem because you become less predictable to yourself. You become less predictable to your own brain. In essence, you become a threat to yourself, and your body's natural response to that is to move less, and to use less power. The brain commands us to use less juice because it believes that you may break, What I have done with him is I have artificially messed up his movement map.

All of your clients are experiencing similar things all of the time. If they are not going through regular joint mobility training and regular vision training, then their bodies are scaring them. Do you feel better?

Alex: "Yes."

Eric: "Let's retest this. Push out again. He is back to normal. Thank you, sir. Can we give him a hand? Are you in an RKC? "

Alex: "No."

Eric: "He's up … he was giving me some good power breathing there whenever he was trying to do the test though."

I have thrown a bunch of stuff at you. I only have a few minutes left. I have given you a little preview of our first level course that starts to introduce all of these concepts. I was overwhelmed by the idea of sharing this information in just an hour and a half because it normally takes me 3 days just to introduce myself.

There is a tremendous amount of information out there right now about the human body that is not being applied. This is true regardless of whether you consider yourself an entrepreneur or a businessperson first and a trainer second.

At the end of the day, you cannot fake competence.
You cannot fake endurance, and you cannot fake competence.

We get away with a ton of stuff in the fitness industry that you cannot get away with in any other industry. There is a great old saying in medicine … 3,000 years ago, a Greek physician said,

"It's the doctor's job to entertain the patient while nature heals them."

That is pretty much how fitness is practiced. Entertainment is awesome because it keeps people coming back, but if you are looking for a way to be different, and you have that mindset that makes you want to be better than everyone else is, then that is what I am here to talk to you about. The information is out there.

We have spent millions of dollars on education and research, as well as thousands upon thousands of research hours personally and with clients. We have hundreds of trainers, and we have a master trainer program.

We have seen thousands of clients around the world, and thousands of athletes. We have seen everyone from every day athletes up to world champions, and what is cool is that they all work the same way. You improve their vision, you improve their vestibular system, you improve their movement, and magical things happen. Their pain gets better. They change as human beings.

You are part of this program, NPE, because you want to be better than everybody else is. You are having a competition here this weekend to determine who is the top guy. Again, I could be all touchy-feely, but as I said, I come from that military martial arts background. I spent a bunch of time working with high-level, elite military units, and the SEALs have an interesting saying whenever they are in BUDS; that is their basic SEAL course that they have to go through to get into the SEALs.

After every evolution, or maybe after dragging a log through the surf, and you get into a boat, and somebody's yelling at you the whole time, and you're miserable and cold, they tell everybody that it pays to be a winner because the team that wins is the only team that gets to rest. It pays to have confidence.

Your Opportunity to Excel

Over time, as you develop your businesses, you have to continue to look for those skill sets to differentiate you. That is really the program that we are going to talk about.

We have a little sheet. Did they get passed out? They are going to pass this out to you right now. I am just going to hold it up. It is an order form for a class that we teach called Essentials of Elite Performance.

This is our 3 day class that we teach as an introduction to our system. On day 1 of the system, we do the movement stuff. What you just saw me do up here with him was jamming the joint, testing the muscles, and all that stuff. This is what we do on day 1 of the training program.

On day 2 of the training program, we start talking about the visual system a little bit more, and we talk about reflexes, as well as how reflexes work in the eyes, and how they work in the inner ear. In addition, we give you some more advanced movement exercises.

On day 3 of the training program, we do a lot of visual testing. In other words, what we have done in this particular course is we have taken our first three levels of certification, which are quite long, and we have condensed them down so that you get level one certification on the first day, level two certification on the second day, and level three certification on the third day.

This is a really, really cool program. We only developed this about 2 years ago. As a teacher, I am very much about the need for competence. I demand a lot from the people that come through our courses. I demand a lot of quality participation. One of the interesting things about our programs is that because I demand that from our master trainers, once you come to one of our certification programs, you can come back for free forever. It is a horrible moneymaking model, I understand that, but at the end of the day, I always tell people that the quality of the practitioner does more for my business than anything else.

The material for this course is covered over a period of 3 days, and the time goes by fast. You can send your staff to it because we have made it extremely inexpensive, and you are getting an amazing deal.

If you are interested in finding out more about what we do, then that is the best place to start because the one thing that we will tell you repeatedly is that in your business, you need a map. If you will remember, everybody raised their hand when I asked how many of you would like to be better trainers, or at least how many of you would like your trainers to be better.

There is an interesting thing that I will share with you, and I only have 1 minute left. In combatives, whenever I teach a course for SWAT teams or whomever, one of the things that we always try to teach them is a system … and the system, while it's based on them individually, is really cool because once they all understand what everyone else is doing, they always know when the other guy is in trouble.

They always know when the other guy is in trouble because they share the same thought process. You are already here studying systemization. You need a system of training that is repeatable and reliable. Those are two hallmarks of science as well as two hallmarks of good business; it always needs to be both repeatable and reliable.

I hope that this was at least though provoking for you. At the very minimum, that is what I need to hear. As I have told you, I am not a sales person. I am a coach, hands down. If you want to be better, then you want to have the most cutting edge information, and you want a lifelong educational process. I can help you with that because that is completely what we are dedicated to as a company.

I would like to thank Sean and everyone else in NPE for having me. Thanks for your time.

Accessing the Video and Audio

If you would rather access the audio and video, go to:
http://www.zhealtheducation.com/neurorevolution

Bonus Interview

Sean Greeley of NPE leading up to Dr. Cobb's presentation conducted the following interview. If you would rather listen to the interview, then the Video and Audio link above is available for you.

Sean: Everybody, welcome. This is Sean Greely and I am back for another NPE audio success CD of the month. Today, I have a great interview for you with Dr. Eric Cobb of Z-Health who is going to share with you a little more about Z-Health in a moment.

To start things up I'll tell you that I recently was in Phoenix and attended their three-day Essentials of Elite Performance training course. It was absolutely a fantastic course. It was one of the best that I have been to in a long time.

We were introduced to Dr. Cobb and Z-Health by our good friends John DuCane from Dragon Door and several others from that organization. It is a pleasure to get to know Z-Health, and to get to know Dr. Cobb. I wanted to share the information really about his organization and his programs with everybody on this call today. Dr. Cobb thanks for being here.

Dr. Cobb: Thanks for the offer. I look forward to talking to you.

What is Z-Health?

Sean: Just to give an introduction, could you give us a brief overview? What is Z-Health?

Dr. Cobb: This is one of the questions that I get all of the time. The joke I make just with the Essentials course is that my elevator speech, unfortunately is about three days long (laughs) because the system is pretty complex, but it's only complex until you really start to get a basic feel for what we're doing.

Let me start off by saying it this way, Z-Health at its most basic level is a human performance system. We are interested in maximizing all the attributes that people have. Whether that be making stronger, fitter, leaner, faster for an athlete et cetera.

What's interesting in that process is we approach all of those attributes through the lens of the nervous system. Z-Health is primarily known for being a neurophysiologically based training system.

That sounds a little intense for a lot of people who don't have maybe a strong neurology background or physiology background. The system has evolved out of a real revolution, if you will, in the understanding of the brain, spinal cord, and reflexes et cetera that has occurred over the last 15 to 20 years.

It's really revolutionizing how we first of all get people out of pain as well as start to make the body comp changes, make them stronger, et cetera. In a very short way, I tell people that Z-Health is a neurophysiologic performance training system. Then, I go on to explain it from there (laughs). Does that help?

Sean: Yes, that's great. That is about as short a description as is possible of the program. We will dig more into that in a little bit, because there is so much that I want to share with our members about Z-Health and what it has to offer.

Before we get into that, let's just ... I'd like to have you share a little bit of your story. You have a tremendous story both as a health care professional, as a former chiropractor, as an entrepreneur and a business owner now with Z-Health. It is an amazing story and I would like to have you share a little bit of that with our members.

Could you start with just telling people a little bit about your background and your evolution as a health care professional?

Dr. Cobb's Background

Dr. Cobb: Normally, when I talk about this I tell people that Z-Health really began for me literally as a kid. The joke I make is that I was born with two interests in life and they eventually evolved into Z-Health. Those two interests were fitness and fighting.

This will be a little bit of a long story so bear with me. The basis of the story is this, whenever I was born, I was one of those kids that you hear about that was born with a lot of strange illnesses and some musculoskeletal birth defects et cetera.

Probably from that I tell people that I'm sure there's some deep psychological survival means. I got involved in martial arts when I was five. In that process, developing as an athlete et cetera, I was a fighter, professional fighter, and I also played national level tennis.

What I tell people is that those experiences for me offered a tremendous amount of pain because of all the other stuff that I had going on with my body. Those experiences drove me into studying physical rehabilitation exercise physiology really trying to figure out ways to be a better athlete, and also how to get out of pain.

When I hit college age, I decided that I was going to be a physician of some kind, and I did my premed stuff. And, because of my martial arts background, I was very firmly rooted in the idea that the body was interconnected. I chose to go an alternative route, and I went into the chiropractic profession.

In that process, it was very interesting. There were a lot of different things that happened while I was in college doing my internship that really brought about the evolution of Z-Health.

Let me explain quickly. One of the issues that I was born with was a genetic disease called Schumer's disease. Basically, whenever you see kids that have this particular disease process going on, by the time that they are in their mid-teens they have a really, really significant thoracic hyperkyphosis.

Really, really hunch back, forehead carriage, rounded shoulders, terrible posture, and that has, it has a lot of impact on pain issues, et cetera. I had that. That was one of the things that I had developed over the years. It was severe.

I had exaggerated it by all the sports, et cetera. I tell people for really the first 25 years of my life or so, I cannot remember a day when there was no pain, shoulder pain, back pain, neck pain, something.

Whenever I went to chiropractic college, I realized right away that the esthetic appearance of this posture was not going to be good for a guy who was supposed to be a back doctor. As soon as I got to the school, I said, You know what? I'm with the posture professionals now. I'm going to really get this stuff sorted out.

I went into very intense therapy between chiropractic manipulations, tremendous amount of soft tissue both a rolfing type of soft tissue work, myofascial release work, et cetera.

I was participating in studies at the time as a subject. We were taking x-rays of my thoracic spine, my neck, et cetera. I was doing a tremendous amount of rehabilitative exercises.

This was a basically a six day a week program I was on. I followed it religiously for over a year. There was no change at all in my body by the end of it. This was incredibly frustrating.

At that point, I said, I'm going to try something different. Interestingly enough, two of my doctors that were overseeing my internship had been to Czechoslovakia and studied with a gentleman named Vladimir Janda. Dr. Janda, if you have any background in medicine and particularly in medicine coming out of the neurology end of things; there are three doctors from Czechoslovakia that are quite well-known and considered the grandfathers of this process. Dr. Janda was one of them.

Janda at that time had developed what he called proprioceptive retraining protocol. A lot of us would recognize that today as unstable surface training. Wobble boards, wobble sandals, a ton of posture corrective work, et cetera because my intern docs had been over there and training with him I had the opportunity to be one of the first people in the US to go through this protocol.

I spent about another nine months learning how to wobble, spin the wobble boards, and move, and on and on and on with different therapy practices. Unfortunately, at the end of that process, there was still no change at all in my posture, and the pain levels were the same.

It was at that point that things began to click for me that I had to try something different because I tell people, I'm always of the mind that if I'm working as hard as I can and the people that I'm working with are also working as hard as they can and we're not seeing the results, then maybe there's something inherently missing within the system that we're applying.

That really was the genesis of Z-Health. It led me to studying a tremendous amount about movement, about posture, about posture correction, whether things are happening consciously or pre-cognitively in the brain in other words; is posture controlled by the spinal cord and the brain stems, almost like breathing, or is it more something that you have to think about?

In that process, I began developing and experimenting with a variety of different exercise protocols, but really with a different focus than I had ever seen before anywhere else. That has fully evolved into this system that we now call Z-Health.

Sean: That is awesome. It's an amazing story, and it's always I don't know, I think we have all these ... what we perceive as obstacles and hurdles in life and things that we get put in front of us. It is only through overcoming them that amazing growth things happen.

In your case, Z-Health is around today because you've gone through all the frustration, trials and tribulations that you have in your own health experience.

25 Years of Pain...Gone!

Dr. Cobb: One of my favorite quotes, I can't remember who it's by right now but it says, *It only took me 10 years to become an overnight success*. (Laughs). That is how I think about this process.

There was a tremendous amount of work that went into it ahead of time to really learn and understand what was happening in my body, and then absolutely what's been happening in athletes' bodies.

I forgot the most important part in my story there, which was that whenever I finally clicked to the idea of the initial stages of Z-Health and really began to focus on precision exercises that were intentionally designed to improve the nervous system functioning.

When I started developing the movements and practicing them, the previous 25 years of pain and posture problems et cetera corrected in about three months. That to me was a phenomenal experience.

Especially talking about what you're saying. It is very interesting to watch people who have gone through different growth processes. I see this in our own business because we have a lot of professionals that we work with.

So many people share similar stories. That is one of the things that I am always trying to get across to our athletes that there is so much about persistence that is so important.

Persistent Application

It's the persistent application in pursuit of your target whatever that is, whether that is better movement, or lean body mass, or making more money. You have to be persistent in that pursuit and just keep altering your approach until you find the path that seems to work for you.

What's cool about that to me is that the more we understand about neurology and understanding some of the basics of Z-Health, the more we realize how much that echoes what is really supposed to happen in the human brain. Every human brain processes information somewhat differently.

It's no surprise for me anymore that people have to shape their own path in building whatever it is that's of interest to them. The biggest predictor is if you are willing to be persistent (laughs) in your tenacity to reach that goal. It has been a very enlightening experience to watch people do physically what they also have to do in their business.

Sean: Absolutely, it just reinforces that the only way you fail is when you quit.

The Only Way to Fail

Dr. Cobb: Yes absolutely. One of my favorite things that interestingly enough in our second level certification we talk a tremendous amount about is the process of motivating or helping people to find motivation because I'm sure that your members know that's one of the biggest challenges that we all face in the health and fitness world. It is this process of being a great coach and having an actual approach to coaching people.

I don't know if you're familiar with the work of a guy named Prochaska. Dr. Prochaska developed a model called the Stages of Change Model. This is basically a psychology approach.

Successfully Making A Change

In essence, I really love it because they did in psychology what we've done in Z-Health, which is they reverse engineered successful people. They said, you know what? Psychology for years and years and years has only focused on looking at people who are sick. They needed professional help somewhere else to make changes in their life.

These people approached it completely differently, and they said, *Let's find a bunch of people who successfully change their own life*. They did this massive study and over 30,000 participated.

What was very interesting is that they went into this process expecting to find very specific change strategies, in other words look at 10,000 people who had successfully lost weight. They were thinking that everyone would probably have a similar strategy.

What they found was that the strategy was different for every single person, but what was consistent was that they went through different stages in the change process.

Ultimately what they came to realize was that the number one predictor of success no matter how many times you quit and had to restart, the number one predictor of success was persistence.

That's something that we're always trying to share with people as well, as we teach these processes in what's called motivational interviewing and motivational coaching, is that our main goal and our main job with all of our clients, with all of our athletes and with ourselves is to continue to find strategies and techniques to just keep you involved in the change process, because if you just stay with it, then good things happen.

Sean: Excellent. Along those lines, I would love for you to share a little bit about your background story as an entrepreneur. As you know, Dr. Cobb, we work with business owners, and so everybody that owns a business is an entrepreneur who has been through different stages of growth and absolutely exercised persistence in becoming successful.

You've got an amazing story in that regard as well. It really is your rise in the chiropractic community, your eventual departure from there, and the growth of Z-Health to what it is today, which is truly remarkable. Would you mind sharing a little bit about your story on the business side of things as well?

Z-Health: The Business

Dr. Cobb: Sure. What I try … I guess when I talk about stuff like this, I tell people that it is probably important to understand a little bit about my personality. I am, because of my fighting background I have, I tell people that I have a very practical personality (laughs).

I want to see results really, really quickly no matter what I'm doing. When I first went to college, I was studying exercise physiology. About two years into that process, I decided that it was not for me because I knew that I did not want to spend my life in a lab. I'm very much results oriented, and I want to see people perform better today.

In that process, as I said, I wound up going to chiropractic college. When I got out of school, I immediately went into practice. It was a very strange and eye-opening experience for me because I realized at that time that very early on I had very strong difficulties or problems with the traditional chiropractic model because I went to the best chiropractic college in the world at the time.

We were receiving a tremendously high-level education in all of the different sciences. It was a very strange process to go through and realize that the actual application, in practice, was very different from what we knew educationally.

I tell people, I was very different from the very beginning. The first day I walked into practice I said to my first new patients, *I'll see you three times. If you're not fixed within three visits, then we're doing something wrong.*

That's not always the case or not always true depending on the level of trauma that they've undergone, but for the most part, as I've learned more and more about neurology, neurophysiology, and pain, it's fairly easy to change pain experiences for people.

I got into practice and I started off working for someone else. After about 6 months I bought a practice. Went in, changed everything, and after several years of being in practice I began to realize that I had moved even further away from the chiropractic model meaning the manipulation, adjustments, and the more passive care were an important piece of the puzzle for acute problems, but I really wasn't fixing people's lives.

The more I was studying neurophysiology at the time, the more I began to realize that long-term impact, long term changes in the body was much more related to lifestyle and teaching people to move well.

In essence, in finding that process, I realized that one of the biggest lacks for me was actually the psychology, the capacity to motivate people, to continue to help and to create change in their own life.

After several years in practice, I had been in that same, during that same time at night and, at work, working on the Z-Health model, building up the full body exercise programs, multiple levels, really researching the neurology of movements or neurology of pain, trying to put into an applicable model and a teachable model.

I sold my practice. At that time, I did something that I had always wanted to do because I said that I would do it; I moved to Italy for a year. I lived in Florence. I had a friend there that was in practice and was working with a lot of the Olympic athletes from Italy.

I moved there, and I worked a couple of days a week with him working with the athletes, and I spent a bunch of time in Tuscany (laughs), which was an amazing experience that I really loved.

After a year, I decided that I was ready to start teaching and moved back to the US, and began literally from scratch, teaching Z-Health. It was also during that time, the other half of my life was also in play. As I mentioned, I was a martial artist. In addition to traditional martial arts, which I only did for a short time, I was really involved in what's called close quarter combat.

I spent a lot of time in this transitional period as well teaching close quarter combat to the military and law enforcement groups as well. That is my volunteer stuff that I do at this point. I work with law enforcement and SWAT teams in the area where I live regularly. That keeps me athletically engaged and that is my community service as well.

Long-term where all of this led, whenever I got back to the states, I initiated the teaching process and training process. That was in 2003; we taught our very first Z-Health course. Seven years later, we have over a thousand people that have gone through different Z-Health courses. We have about 600 certified.

We have an institute, multiple level certifications, and a master training program as well. We just opened up about an 8,000 square foot facility last year in Phoenix, Arizona because that's where ... we do work with a lot with professional athletes at this point, and they like to travel to where it's sunny.

We're continuing to see tremendous growth. I teach most of the certification courses; I probably teach 90% of the certification courses myself still at this point because I really love to teach. It is one of my favorite things to do. The only issue with that is I travel about 220 days a year because we do teach all around the country.

About a year and a half ago, I moved internationally as well and I am teaching in Europe and I am supposed to be headed to Australia this year.

Sean: It's a tremendous story, and I know that in many ways this has been 7 years in the making, but now you're starting to really hit full strides with Z-Health. I have no doubt that those numbers will double and triple very quickly here as the early adapters like myself, I'm always an early adapter kind of guy, start to get the word out to others about this amazing program, really just what it has to offer, which is tremendous.

We're going to get more to that in just a second. Let's transition now and ... would you share one of your long-term goals of Z-Health?

Long-term Z-Health Goals

Dr. Cobb: I can try to sum it up in a pretty easy statement, although it sounds grandiose when I say it. You have to forgive me. We really see Z-Health long-term as a system that is helping to initiate what I consider a revolutionary approach to working with the human body.

Z-Health actually fits the legal definition of a new profession because of all the different pieces that we pull in. Most of the practitioners that come to us at this point are either in the fitness industry or in the health care industry. Z-Health is as a system and as a profession, bridging the gap between the two.

Our long-term goals are to make inroads into every field that deals with the human body because the more that we understand about neurology, the more we're learning that you really can't separate psychology from physiology. We now are actually getting psychologists who are using Z-Health with their clients and their patients.

We have trainers who are studying motivation. We have vision specialists who are now studying movements. In many ways, we are a system that allows professionals to fill in the missing pieces of the puzzle to what they are currently doing.

You mentioned the term early adapters, which I really appreciate because that really describes the people that are currently involved in Z-Health, who have the vision to say you know what? We have learned more in the last 10 or 15 years about neurology and neurophysiology than we have in all of history. That is a huge deal.

Are You Staying Current?

I tell people that if you want to stay current in business, then you want to make a lot of money in the next 15 years doing things that are tremendously helpful for people. You have to begin to understand their neurology and a term that is called neuroplasticity, which means that the brain could change, and it can learn and grow at any age, which is really a different thought process than those people are used to have in medicine.

We see ourselves as a long-term goal, as a system that is going to help bridge the gap between fitness in the health care industry and over time separate Z-Health out as a separate profession.

It is very interesting to watch our high level trainers and our master trainers work with clients because in a single session you may see them specifically teaching a lot of exercise stuff because that's what we do, and that's what we're known for.

In that process, we're using exercise to help people to maybe improve pains, or maybe in the same session they're working with an athlete improving their sports skill.

They may be improving that sports skill by working with their eyes or working with their balance system, their inner ear, or something within their joints. It is fascinating to watch all the tools being implemented. That is one major goal, as I said; it is going to bridge the gap between these systems.

Number two, my other really long-term goal is to actually see a Z-Health type curriculum instituted in the public school setting. One of the things that I feel really strongly about is youth programs, youth physical development, and youth movement development, because society seems to be promoting less and less movement.

Poor health, the obesity issue as we all know is reaching epidemic proportions. People are becoming less and less athletic. I believe that is an unnatural state. So, I am trying to teach kids from a very early age how to move, and how to stay athletic for their whole life because I think that long-term it has a tremendous impact on us as a society.

Sean: Absolutely, those are tremendous goals. I know that, at least what I have seen so far I know that you are well on your way. Let's give folks a little more breakdown overview of Z-Health and what it involves.

Would you mind explaining the different certifications that you offer, and give people a little bit of an overview of the different types of certifications you offer and how the program is laid out to progress people through all the things that they need, the tools they need, to help people to get out of pain and improve their life.

Z-Health's Certification Courses

More about Z-Health Courses

Dr. Cobb: Sure. I will try to do this really succinctly. The very first course that we recommend people to come to because we consider it a pre-certificating course is called Essentials of Elite Performance.

It's a three-day course; on day one we cover material from level one certification, on day two we cover materials from our level two certification, and on day three we cover materials from our level three certification. It is a great introduction to the system and it really gives people an overview of Z-Health as well as what it has to offer.

With that said, let me discuss our certifications. We have four basic certifications, level one is called R-Phase; the R stands for rehabilitation. A lot of people hear that and shy away. However, they should not because when you look at every athlete you have ever worked with whether that is a pro athlete or an office-worker athlete, they all have stuff that needs to be fixed.

R-Phase is really about helping people to understand neurophysiology in a very practical level as well as understanding how important it is to constantly be assessing and reassessing clients. We teach gate assessments, we teach range of motion assessments, and we teach several other things within that course in a very unique way.

We also teach you a movement tool box, including how to train the nervous system through joint specific movements. There are 160 drills that we teach within that particular course as well as when to apply them and how to apply them.

The second course, the second certification is called I-Phase; the I stands for integration. I-Phase is a lot more athletic movement patterns; we really begin talking about how your vision and your inner ear or your vestibular system affects movement.

We teach you very simple assessments to look at your client's visual system and their vestibular system to see if maybe this is impacting on that lousy shoulder range of motion, or their back pain, or the fact that they can't squat. We have a very *find it, fix it* approach in both of those courses.

Level three certification is called S-Phase, which is sports skill. One of the things that I love about that course is that it is really subdivided into different components; one is a movement component.

In the movement component, we teach the basics of sports movement. Do you know how to sprint? Do you know how to cut? Do you know how to turn, like a high-level athlete?

One of the things that I've been frustrated about for years and years and years is that many people give up sports or never start sports because no one teaches them how to move like an athlete. They are always behind their competitors, which is a poor motivational process.

We teach the basics of sports movement, and that's an amazing process in and of itself, to have clients safely learning how to run, how to sprint, how to cut, how to stop at any age. It really opens up the doors for people to have tremendously different but highly effective training sessions; it makes you unique.

The second part of that course is a much greater exploration of the visual system where we teach you basic tools from what's called Behavioral Optometry. This is still all within licensure of a fitness professional so that's really cool.

It allows you to really look at how are people's eyes working? Are they appropriate for life? Are they appropriate for their sport? One of the things that you oftentimes find is that people are not athletic, not because they cannot move, but because their eyes are interfering with their movement. Assessments and drills can fix things within that environment.

T-Phase, which is our 4th level certification, is for those people who are really interested in dealing with pain, or need a hands-on work for athletes. It is called Therapy Phase.

Most of the people that attend that course are not therapists, they're not licensed to be therapists, and they don't need to be to practice any of the material that we teach in the course.

One of the things that we try to make people understand is that if you're a fitness professional, then you have to have the knowledge of pain. You also have to have a knowledge of what to do with it whether that's to refer it out or to be able to help people quickly to deal with it and get them back into training. That is what course is focused on.

Following those four certifications, people then have the opportunity to enter our Mater Trainer program, which is an additional year program that really enforces high quality or high-level expertise with all the material out of the four courses. Our Master Trainers are now producing products under our brand, teaching for us and traveling for us. That has been an incredibly exciting process.

Finally, on top of all of that, we also offer specialty courses from our fitness model, which is called the 9S model; 9S' of fitness. We teach specialty courses and special certifications.

The one that we did last year was called Sustenance meaning food and nutrition but really the substance of the course had a tremendous amount of psychology in it as well as how to coach people from a motivational perspective on diet.

We consider the Z-Health program a lifelong educational model because there is so much information in all the courses. We know that it takes time, but we really establish relationships with everyone that attends our courses, and we look forward to working with them permanently, because we consider Z-Health a lifelong educational process. I am always learning and our master trainers are always learning.

We try to build that kind of culture in the Z-Health that once you initiate the process, we're with you for the long-term because we believe that it's the ongoing educational process that gives you a competitive advantage that sets you apart from the crowd that's out there teaching fitness or teaching or working in health care facilities et cetera.

Sean: It sounds like …

Dr. Cobb: I hope I didn't take two hours.

Sean: Yes, no, that was a great, I picture that, and you knocked it out of the park. That was a great description of what you have to offer in a condensed explanation. I will just share with folks that when I attended the Essentials course, which is what I absolutely recommend to all of our folks. You should go check it out when you can get to one, and if there's one coming in your area. Even if there is none, take a few days off, fly out to a course, and take the time to go through it.

The Essentials was an absolutely amazing experience. I saw several folks there that I talked to and met over there over the 3 day course that had been to other of your programs, and they were coming back again.

It seems very much that your values are in educating and working with your members, and that it's a lifelong process; it is very much the same as the way we work with our folks, and the relationship that we have with our customers; a lot of things in alignment there. That just it's fun to see and it's fun to get to know each other.

Let's transition and talk, we'll just keep going on here. I would like to have you address what brings someone out to a training session. Why does somebody come to a Z-Health course?

Why Attend A Z-Health Course?

Dr. Cobb: If I'm very honest about this, then the one word that I have to choose is dissatisfaction. That may strike people as odd, but the reason that I say that is generally when people come to a new course or new event of any kind, they are there because they do not feel like their model is quite set yet.

If we were completely happy with the results we were getting, if we were completely happy with the money we were making, then most people at that point get comfortable and they don't continue to look for new information. I have to say that there is some level of dissatisfaction, number one.

Secondly, you've already mentioned another important word, which was early adopter. People that come out to a Z-Health course are legitimately interested in making a difference in people's lives. They are looking for a faster, more efficient system to make that happen. They are definitively looking for cutting-edge information.

The people that attend our courses typically have been in the industry long enough to fit into the category that I have mentally of a real professional. Someone who understands that mastery of his or her craft requires time, it requires effort, it requires money, and it requires an ongoing focus of being better.

That's really a perfect description of people that show up at Z-Health courses. We don't get very many folks showing up who've done maybe a two or three days fitness certification, or who have been involved in the industry for two or three months. That is not our demographic.

Our demographic includes business owners who are trying to set apart their company or their business from their competitors by having a strong competitive advantage with regards to results.

The other thing that I will say is that people are also drawn to Z-Health particularly out of the fitness industry because much of what we teach has an immediate, observable impact on performance and pain as well as range of motion issues.

I'm very clear on this with people from the very beginning because there are people in the fitness industry who would argue that if a client is in pain, then that really is the doctor's realm.

Realistically if we had to refer out every single client, every single time because they were in pain, then no one would be training because 95% of people when you ask them, "Is something bothering you?" They will go, "Yes, my knee, my shoulder, my ankle."

Part of our educational process is starting to help people to recognize that it's really easy to help most people through appropriate exercise, appropriate mobility work, maybe visual work, or maybe inner ear work, whatever to get out of pain very quickly in a very safe manner.

That's another reason that people come to Z-Health, we have a reputation for helping people to get out of pain very quickly, and helping them to restore a range of motion very quickly.

You get someone who can't raise their right arm, or who can't move their left foot, or their left knee, or whatever. Most of that stuff is pretty easy, and so that's another reason that people show up because they're looking for tools to really improve their clients workout. if I can say it that way, because as we all know, when you've got the client that walks in and they really can't raise their right arm, they're not going to get much of a workout.

They'll show up if we're doing a good job interviewing them, but as far as creating that long-term result and change, one of the things that I'm always talking about with our trainers is to listen to every client that you have. This is a walking billboard for you and for the service that you provide.

You need to have skills to make them look like the billboard that you want walking around. I think that professionals who already have that deep realization are the ones that seek out our courses.

Sean: I'll just add to that that really for the folks that are committed to getting the best results possible for their clients whether that is through themselves, or through their staff, the Z-Health is a program that can absolutely improve your game, head and shoulders above what you're doing today, because this information is truly groundbreaking.

I haven't learned about it anywhere else, and I've never seen anybody put it together in a format that you have. It is truly unique. This is true whether you are working with high performance athletes, or folks that are in pain, or just ordinary folks that you want to help to get better results faster, across the board in every area and a measure of health and fitness as well as life improvement. Z-Health will benefit you and benefit your organization. You have a saying about the top 1%. Do you want to mention that?

Z-Health's Charter

Dr. Cobb: Yes. We have talked a little bit about the business building aspect, and the entrepreneurial aspect. In describing Z-Health, whom we work with, and what we say is our primary goal. Our company charter is to train the top 1% in any field.

Most people say, "Well, Doc shouldn't that be the top 1% in the health and fitness field?" Realistically, the answer is no because we have had a number of people go through our certifications who really are not fitness professionals, but instead are in other arenas like psychology.

We are now, interestingly enough, getting high-level execs, maybe project managers, et cetera. We have had several Microsoft professionals coming into the course because they have had friends that went through it. And, they've said that understanding how human physiology works as well as how the brain works has made them tremendously more effective even in their fields, which to me makes perfect sense because realistically everything we do is driven by our neurology.

Our system is about having a deep understanding of that. Our company charter is to train the Top 1%. We say that unapologetically because we believe that people that are in the top 1% of their field are the industry changers. They are the world changers.

We feel strongly enough about our product and our system that those are the people that we want to work with. Our course has changed literally every two to three months based off interactions, and based off research.

In essence, what we're doing in the Z-Health community is building a highly talented master mind group, if I can call it that, because as we are all working together towards this common goal of the unifying lens of how we look at the body. We are seeing an evolution in the process of fitness training, health care, et cetera.

As an example, and this one is fascinating because it just popped up for me about two days ago. In our level four course (T-Phase), two and a half years ago, we introduced the concept from a neurophysiologic concept called the Threat Neuromatrix. This fancy sounding term explains a lot about neurophysiology as well as how the brain and body react to our environment.

We've been using this term for quite some time, and just last week someone forwarded me a letter to the editor of The Pain Practice, which is one of the major pain journals in the world. There was a letter to the editor, someone has taken our concept and now he is saying that we are proposing that pain research in general be reclassified using the term Threat Neuromatrix, et cetera.

This stuff is really exciting to me to see that our concepts are showing up around the world in different fields. As I said, that top 1% concept is very important to me because when you surround yourself with other likeminded individuals, which is what you are promoting through NPE, it makes a tremendous difference in your capacity to learn number one things that work as well as things that don't work.

Number two is just to have that external motivation, if you will, of being around people who are excellent. That is our primary goal in that.

Sean: I'd like to break down a little bit more for folks about the Essentials training. That is the program that I attended at Phoenix for 3 days, and I just had a tremendous experience going through the course.

I'll share with you that this stuff I've seen it and I believe it. If someone had told me about some of the benefits that people can experience in Z-Health, I listen but I really have to see it to believe it.

I can vouch for that now. I went through some different drills. I did a test, the flexibility test, or strength test, and then I did a few more drills. Literally, a minute later, I got another 10 to 15 degrees range of motion in a joint, or testing almost 50% higher on a strength test in a minute just from doing a couple of drills.

It's really wild, and it's unbelievable just to talk about it; it would have been hard for me to accept that if I hadn't seen it. I just encourage you to check it out when you get the chance to check out the Essentials course, because it's amazing.

I actually got to spend more time working with Dr. Cobb privately after the 3 days course, and he gave me a regimen to work on to improve, as well as get some of my own benefits that I can out of Z-Health. I have been working through that and I am continuing to see improvement as a result.

Could you break down the Essentials course? What are those 3 days, and what does it look like for the folks who attend that program?

The Essentials of Elite Performance

More about the Essentials course

Dr. Cobb: Day one is, as I said, R-Phase. And, in day one we spend quite a bit of time explaining the basics of neurophysiology as we currently understand them, as well as helping people to understand how movement is formed in the nervous system, and then making a really strong argument for helping people to understand why we teach some of the drills that we teach and why we teach them the way that we do.

I tell people that all exercise is a vehicle that speaks to the nervous system. We have to train the nervous system enough to make it adapt, but if we overdo it, then we're going to see it not adapt like we want.

Day one is really about beginning a process of cleaning up movement, and also helping people to understand how quickly their body changes when we know what to look for. We are very big on teaching immediate reassessment.

One of the things that I get really frustrated about in watching health and fitness professionals is that there is a lot of guessing that goes on. The guessing, I guess I will say this, I will try to say it in a nice way; it is not an intentional desire to guess.

Whenever you've been taught assessments over the course of the years without really a focus on reassessments and understanding how fast the body changes, most people are shooting in the dark, based off of a biomechanical concept or a biomechanical model.

The thing that has happened over the course of the last 15 years is we've come to understand that there's a tremendous amount of limitation with the biomechanical model. Let me give you a perfect example.

About a month ago, we were in the UK in London South Hampton area, South Bank area. We were at a sports university there teaching the Essentials course. One of the gentlemen that arrived at the course was an exercise physiology professor from Germany.

On a break, I was asking him why he was there, and we were talking a little bit. He said, *I've seen some very interesting things about Z-Health online, and I've played around with some of the drills because I bought the product. They made a big difference for me, but I really do not have a great rationale for it. What I'm here to have is a rationale.*

Hey! I Can Raise My Arms!

I said, "Do you have anything really major going on with your body?" He said, "Yes, let me show you." He had limited internal rotation of his right shoulder, and almost no internal rotation of his right shoulder.

He had had it for about seven years, and he had been told that he had a labral tear and frozen shoulder, and capsular adhesions, and then they said that he needed surgery, and he declined the surgery. He had just been living with it.

As an example, I am going to move ahead into day three really quickly. We did some physical work from day one, R-Phase, we gave him some mobility drills, and it made some difference, but what made a tremendous difference for him was actually his visual system.

In fact, we gave him one visual drill from day three of the Essentials course. And, in the space of 60 seconds of doing the eye work, he got full range of motion back in his right shoulder.

That is a thing that we see every day in the health that's coming, that's why we're talking about things that are seemingly unbelievable until you've seen it a bunch of times.

I am saying all that as a reminder for day one that we are trying to help people get out of the biomechanical mindset. Day one is this paradigm shift from biomechanical things into neurologic thinking.

On day two, which is the I-Phase part of the course, we talk about your eyes and your inner ear. We teach you more advanced movement drills, but really, this whole day is about helping people to understand that when the visual system is messed up, the vestibular system is messed up, and your movement will never be as good as it could be. You will typically always have little pain issues that are arising, et cetera.

We teach simple assessments and drills for the visual system and the vestibular system. On day three, which I've already mentioned, we teach more visual drills, more visual assessments, and also begin to introduce people to the basics of sports and athletic training.

One of the things that I always find fascinating on day three is that I have everybody in the course and probably I will say, "Raise your hand if you're an athlete." We usually have about a 90% rate where people raise their hands and they said yes, I play tennis, or soccer, or football, or whatever.

I ask a simple question, "How many of you played it through college?" Normally, about 30% will still have their hands up. I'm starting to identify the elite athletes if you will or people who have played at a higher level.

I ask a simple question, "How many of you in all of your sports training were ever taught how to sprint? How many of you were taught how to cut?" Usually, one person at most will have their hand up.

I always point that out as a great example of the mistakes that we tend to make, people in the health and fitness industry, particularly the strength and conditioning industry go, everybody just needs to get stronger and I say, "No you need to get better."

Day 3 is really about helping people to learn the basics of athleticism. It is amazing. I love day 3 because I see the light bulbs come on so often for fitness professionals who begin to realize that there are so many different ways that they can work with their clients day-to-day in an exciting, interesting way that's about skill building, and really helping people to build a more athletic body map as well as a more athletic picture of themselves.

That's, I like to say that day 3 is always very exciting for me as well. That is the three-day course in a nutshell. It is a very fast course, very fast paced. The days go really quickly.

Most of the courses are about half lecture, half movement. And, as I said... what I really enjoy about the course is the people that attend it have done tremendously well in our certification programs. Helping them to get that early vision of the Z-Health system as a whole seems to make the whole difference for their capacity to apply it day-to-day.

Sean: That's a great overview of the Essentials program, and I'm glad that you shared the story of the gentleman from the UK, which is the one that you shared during the week when I was present.

It actually made me think about here is a guy seven years, no range of motion, and the doctors are all telling him that he's got to have surgery but he avoids it because he is an exercise physiologist and he doesn't want to succumb to that. Within a few drills in a couple of days he's got 100% range of motion back, which I can only imagine what that must have felt like.

If you can't move your arm for seven years, and then all of a sudden you got the thing back 100%, it's absolutely amazing. As you said, those stories are very, very common with Z-Health students. I am wondering if you could just share a couple more client success stories like that, that you have seen or experienced having gone through the training.

Some Cool Results

Dr. Cobb: I'll give you, we have, and again this is not to say that I'm overly up on the Z-Health system because I love it as my system. I am still fascinated by how well it works, if I can say it that way. We have hundreds of success stories if not thousands on file.

I'll tell you a couple of ones that still stick in my head simply because they were so cool. About two years ago one of our trainers, we were teaching in southern, sorry in northern California. He asked me to look at the husband of one of his clients.

I said, "Hey, what's going on?" They set up this appointment. It was funny to me because it was like every other time that you have ever had anyone come to you very begrudgingly.

It is the wife dragging the husband, and I could tell that he did not want to be there. I sat down with them, and right away, I tried to build some rapport. I said, "Tell me your story."

His story was really horrific. For no reason that they knew of, he had developed bilateral frozen shoulder. This was almost 7 years old at this point. He had maybe 30 degrees of flexion on the right arm, and maybe 40 or 50 on his left arm. He had ongoing pain. He could not raise his arm above that position, and the worst part was that he was a barber.

He had to redesign his workstation because he actually could not raise his arms high enough to even work in the chair. He had been to about six or seven different orthopedics, including a couple of orthopedics for NBA teams.

They all told him that this is one of the worst cases of frozen shoulder that we've seen. You need surgery. They do what was called a closed reduction on a frozen shoulder, which is a pretty brutal process. For some reason, he opted not to do this procedure. He just figured that he would rather deal with the lack of range motion than go through that procedure.

They brought him in to see me. I took his history, checked him out, watched him walk, and did our usual R-Phase assessment. All that I did was... this is the crazy cool part. Watching him walk he had really bad feet, very, very poor mobility in his feet, and very poor joint function.

Most people, when they see bad feet, they think that they need shoes or products. We are completely different. We say that when you have bad feet, you need to have better feet.

We need to improve mobility; we need to improve strength because most of our posture and movement is initiated based on nerve endings coming as well as information coming from nerve endings and the feet.

Long story short, I did three drills with him on his right foot, and three drills on his left foot. *It took less than three minutes to get full range of motion in both shoulders.*

Watching the guy so fired up was amazing. The reason that I remember it though is because he was very non-talkative, and he was really, really happy. I was still at the same facility the next day, I was working with the clients, and I had something at the corner of my eye.

I looked up and I saw him. He stepped around the corner, he smiled at me, he raised both arms all the way up to the ceiling, waved, and then he walked out. He did not say anything else.

He is always stuck in my mind because it was such a huge change and particularly because of the profession. That is an example of a foot drill or a foot and ankle drill of changing shoulder range of motion again, which is very, very common.

Here is another interesting example, but I will not tell you the names, we had an Olympic athlete that was just competing in Vancouver. I was introduced to this athlete because of a serious injury; he was a snowboarder, he had a bad fall, and he had not really been riding the same for over a year.

He just felt like his core did not contract well, that his abdominals were not turning on, and that his musculature was not right. Nothing felt coordinated. I had two sessions with this particular athlete; on the first session, because they had some head trauma, in pieces, we teach how to evaluate the head and neck, and the cranial system, et cetera.

We did some visual drills, we did some cranial mobilization, as well as some stuff with the feet, and we did the same thing the second session. This athlete went back to training, in preparation for the Olympics, and in the space of one week the coaches came back and said, "I have no idea what you've just done but you're riding better than we've ever seen you ride." That was after a year of struggling.

Those are two examples of a head problem fixing coordination, an abdominal coordination issue, a foot problem, and shoulder problems. The drills fix shoulder problems. It is commonplace.

The reason that I bring them out is that I think people find them very intriguing when you talk about, when you hear stuff like that because it resonates on a very deep level with people that the body is more integrated and interconnected than most people believe. That resonates with us intuitively.

What Z-Health offers is a rationale, an actual physiologic, neurologic rationale for why the foot might affect the shoulders, why the skull might affect the abs.

On top of that rationale, we give you assessments and drills to figure out exactly what needs to happen in order to help your clients succeed. I could go on and on with different stories about eyes changing movement, about inner ear work changing movement, but hopefully those are a couple of neat examples. If you want more, then you can always call and talk to us. There is plenty.

Sean: That is great. I appreciate you sharing that. I wanted you to share some of the stories because it really illustrates the power of the human body as well as this paradigm shift in health and fitness care. By moving to the Z-Health model, which is more neurologically based in the prescription, we see immediate results. The traditional paradigm might take months and years to see results.

You are proving that is not the reality. Rather you see it as a body responds to the speed of the nervous system, which is, as you taught us in our course, that it goes at 300 miles per hour.

Dr. Cobb: 300 miles an hour.

Sean: Yes. Within a few seconds, the body can change dramatically when you learn to understand that and start to apply some of these principles, and drills, and exercise into care. It is something that I ... again it's a pleasure to do this interview today because the word just needs to continue to get out there for folks.

If you have been struggling with any issues with your own health or fitness, or just want to constantly improve as many of our folks are high performers, or the clients that you work with that your traditional programming just is not getting the same results.

You are committed to continue to improve your own programming and models of providing care to your clients as well as improving performance.

This is something that you need to learn more about and integrate into your practice.

With that being said, I would like to just wrap this up here and give some folks information on how to find out more about Z-Health and about how to find information about an upcoming essentials course that may be coming in their area or one that they could get to. Could you give folks the details on how to get that information?

Dr. Cobb: Yes, absolutely. The easiest way to find out more about us, without talking to a lot of human beings, is to go to our website that's zhealth.net. There is no hyphen or anything; it is just zhealth.net. On that website, you will find all of our courses listed and our calendar, as well as descriptions of our certifications and our products, et cetera.

From there, we also really urge you to call our office. We love to talk to people in person. Things have become very depersonalized. We want to answer your questions.

Our toll free number is 888-394-4198. You can call and speak to any of our staff.

Finally, if you want to email us, then you can email us at info@zhealth.net and we will get right back to you to answer your questions.

If this is something that you are interested for yourself or for your clients, then you should make sure to call us so that we can talk to you and tell you some of the special things that we have. Because I will say that we've been very impressed with what you are doing, and with the focus on building that top 1%.

I always tell people when I am teaching about these courses to listen and be selfish first in this particular case. Every fitness professional that I know has some nagging injury or nagging problem that they need to take care of at a basic level. We want to start with you because Sean and I appreciate the fact that you said that you have to see it to believe it, and most people do.

We would love to have you get to an Essentials course, or to meet up with a high level trainer or master trainer in your facility or your area as possible, just so you can start to experience what we do.

Sean: Dr. Cobb thanks again for this interview today. I really appreciate it and it is a pleasure getting to know you and your organization, as well as starting to work together here.

Dr. Cobb: Thanks very much for your time. I enjoyed talking with you.

If you would rather access the audio and video, go to:

http://www.zhealtheducation.com/neurorevolution

Made in the USA
Las Vegas, NV
09 January 2023

65311087R00068